I0483967

Practical Behavioural Handbook for Paediatric Clinics

Professor Ashoka Jahnavi Prasad

Copyright © 2015 Professor Ashoka Jahnavi Prasad

Dedicated to Jaya and Ajai ,two of the most dedicated paediatricians I know.

Table of Contents

Interrupting others during conversations (phone or face to face)

Morning routine for school days

Parent Journal of Treatment Progress: Morning Routine

Parent Handouts for each Treatment Package (can be posted for easy

viewing)

Going to bed on time

Night waking (The Cipani Proximity-fading

Method) Nighttime accidents
Sibling rivalry at home

Car trips (The Cipani tolerance training

method) Following rules of playground

Putting up toys after play The "Cipani 3 toy rule" Interrupting

others during conversations (phone or face to face) Morning

routine for school days

Preface

Clinicians (pediatricians, mental health professionals, family physicians) who serve families are regularly presented with parental complaints about child behavior management problems that involve certain settings, daily activities, or time periods. For example, various bedtime problems are a frequent behavioral pediatric concern expressed by parents. Some parents report difficulty in getting their child to bed at a reasonable time. The form of child problem behaviors during this time can range from minor complaining for a protracted period of time (complaints about not wanting to go to bed) to more disruptive attempts to escape going to bed (such as extreme tantrums and disruptive behavior). Another common problem concerns their child's disruptive episode upon waking up at night.

Ten common behavioral pediatric problem areas are represented in this clinical resource. Each area is addressed with a treatment package approach. Each treatment package provides a number of parenting tips and suggestions (i.e., components) that form the basis of the clinical intervention for that particular area. Some families may have problems in multiple areas. It is suggested that if there are multiple problem areas, that the clinician address one problem area at a time. Each tip is explained in terms of its relationship to the solution of the problem, and is written from the perspective of the parent reading the material.

This resource material for clinicians is comprised of behaviorally-based solutions to such problems. It aims to solve such problems through the clinician teaching the parents how to more effectively manage the particular circumstance. The suggestions offered comprise a parental repertoire that deals more effectively with the circumstance. Many of the treatment components come from the research literature in applied behavior analysis. While not every family will respond to such a treatment package with positive results (even if such procedures are carried out with integrity), the research literature supports the deployment of parent training as an efficacious clinical treatment strategy for many families.

The model used for this behavioral approach is one of consultation with parents. The parents will play a pivotal role in the solving of the particular problem. Therefore, a substantial amount of the "therapy time" should be spent reviewing each recommendation with the parent(s) and how such can be put into practice in their specific circumstance. There are also data sheets that should form the basis of the clinician's monitoring of the child's progress in the particular problem area during weekly therapy sessions with the parents. In most cases, the parents should be encouraged to deploy all the components of the treatment package in order to possibly realize a significant behavioral effect for that particular problem area.

Clinicians will also find the format of the material for each problem area useful as handouts to parents (each of the ten areas also has a one-sheet handout in the back for easy posting on the refrigerator or wall if desired by the parent).

———————————————

Eating too much

1.

In many cases, the problem with children who eat too much is the number and amount of snacks they are afforded (or obtain by other means). If you believe your child needs a snack, you should schedule a healthy snack and require some effort to earn it. If needed, a nutritionist can help with your meal plan for your child. **You should also consult with your physician on a reasonable projected weight loss program for your child prior to starting this program.** *Trying to make weight loss occur rapidly can be dangerous, and should not be considered.* Missing meals is not wise and can be dangerous for children. A reasonable (and consistent) loss of weight is preferred.

2. Designate a child-size portion for each meal.

Does your child take huge portions during mealtime? In addition to possibly designating smaller portions for the meal, a new rule to institute is no seconds! When your child is done with the meal, have him or her immediately walk away from the table. In effect, remove temptation to fill the plate again. It would be helpful if there is an engaging planned activity for your child immediately after mealtime.

3. Slow down the rate of eating.

Does your child eat quickly? Slowing down the rate of eating can bolster the desired result to eat less. By slowing down the rate of spoon to mouth, many people find that it reduces the amount of food they eat at any given meal. To accomplish this, after each bite or spoonful, your child should put down the utensil. Have your child count to 10 and then proceed to take another bite or spoonful. Additionally, after every five bites or spoonfuls, have your child drink a little bit of water or other liquid (one with few calories).

4. Activity rewards for weight loss.

Having your child get on a weight scale periodically is a good way to monitor weight loss (or gain). In addition to the above three recommendations, it might be helpful if your child is weighed one to two times a week, and such information is posted on a chart (like a calendar) in plain sight. Setting weekly weight loss goals in collaboration with your physician is a good start, but it needs followthrough. Having a special weekend activity conditional upon achieving the target weight loss for that week could be very helpful (read Section IV in free downloadable ebook, Punishment on Trial, for further information on arranging consequences). **It is strongly advised to have your physician plan, monitor, and follow-up with your child's weight loss.** Ask your physician how frequently he or she would like to monitor your child's weight loss. It is imperative that a reasonable weight loss program for your child be designed and supervised by your physician. Rapid weight loss can be dangerous for children!

Going to bed on time

1. *Setup a consistent schedule for bedtime.*

In many cases, children who have difficulty going to bed on time have no consistent bedtime. Therefore, an essential first step in getting control over bedtime problems is a bedtime schedule. You need to designate a consistent schedule for bedtime for both weekdays and weekends. In fact, to facilitate learning appropriate bedtime behavior, you might initially have the same schedule for all seven days.

2. *A pre-bed routine is necessary.*

The pre-bed routine should end in the child being in his or her bed at the designated time. Here is a sample pre-bed routine. At 8:00 p.m., a seven-year-old child brushes his or her teeth, gets a drink of liquids (*nothing with caffeine*) and uses the toilet. The child then goes to his or her bedroom, puts on pajamas and gets in bed by 8:25 p.m. This sequence of activities within the pre-bed routine should remain the same, *especially* during the first 6-8 weeks.

3. *Bedtime stories are conditional upon being in bed on time.*

Many children love to have bedtime stories read to them. You can use this to your advantage in solving bedtime problems. In the above scenario, the child was to be in bed at 8:25 p.m. If the child is in bed at or before 8:25 p.m., the child earns a bedtime story. However, if the child is not in bed by 8:26 p.m., then he or she goes to bed without a story. The length of story time should be fixed with a timer to avoid arguments about how long you should read (have a timer by the bedside for this reason).

4. *After the bedtime story, no other competing activities should occur in the bed.*

If you are going to teach your child to fall asleep upon going to bed, you cannot allow them to watch TV or play video games once in bed. Those activities would interfere with the development of a quick sleep onset pattern (this is also true for adults who have difficulty with sleep onset).

5. *A bedtime pass is provided if the child gets to bed by the designated time.*

In addition to earning the bedtime story, the child also earns a bedtime pass that allows him or her to leave the bed just once for any additional need. The bedtime pass was developed by Dr. Pat Friman and fellow researchers at the University of Kansas, who found it very effective in reducing behavior problems. The bedtime pass is surrendered by the child to allow one trip out of the bed. The child is not allowed to leave the bed subsequently. If the child leaves the bed after the pass is surrendered, an additional consequence is warranted.

6. *A star chart system for adherence is strongly advocated.*

Highly preferred weekend activities can be exchanged for points earned by going to bed on time and not getting up after the bedtime pass has been surrendered. For example, each night that Billy (hypothetical child) gets to bed on time and does not leave the bed subsequent to surrendering his pass, he earns one star. If he earns five stars (out of seven in a week), he gets a designated weekend privilege.

When Billy does not earn at least five stars, the designated weekend privilege is not available for that particular weekend. Of course, every week brings a new opportunity for your child to earn that weekend privilege (read Section IV in free downloadable ebook, *Punishment on Trial,* for further information on arranging consequences). You should track this weekly information on a calendar (or other data sheet such as the one below) to review progress.

Bedtime Star Chart:

If child went to bed and stayed (using bedtime pass only once), place a star on that date

SUN	MON	TUES	WED	THURS	FRI	SAT
Date:	Date:	Date:	Date:	Date:	Date:	Date:
Date:	Date:	Date:	Date:	Date:	Date:	Date:
Date:	Date:	Date:	Date:	Date:	Date:	Date:
Date:	Date:	Date:	Date:	Date:	Date:	Date:

Night waking
(The Cipani Proximity-fading Method)

1. *If your child is not initially falling asleep in their own bed without you, that could contribute to the difficulty.*

> If you allow your young child to fall asleep on the couch next to you, that is setting up the "going to sleep" condition as one which requires your presence. You may need to start putting your child in their own bed (i.e., to fall asleep) as a later part of this program (once tumultuous night wakings have been solved).

2. *Ignoring works but is hard in practice.*

> When young children cry out at night for attention, they want their parent(s) to come to their bed. I am sure you've heard that ignoring such attention-getting behavior is the way to go. Ignoring this behavior is theoretically sound but logistically difficult (if not impossible) in some households. If your child is capable of crying and whining in the middle of the night for 45 minutes or longer, your attempt to ignore such behavior will result in other people waking up and creating havoc. I believe my approach delineated below is more suitable. My colleagues and I have used it in clinical practice with referrals for such problems as crying and tantrums upon waking up at night (we are talking about children, of course). *Especially if you have tried ignoring these incidents of night waking and have been unsuccessful, this plan is for you.* If you believe you can be successful at ignoring the behavior at nighttime, then all power to you.

3. *Go to the child immediately, but do not get in his or her bed.*

Do not allow the child to cry incessantly before you go to his or her bed. In fact, teach the child that simply saying "Mommy, I am up" is sufficient to bring you. This should have the effect of quickly ameliorating lengthy and intense tantrums to get your attention and presence at nighttime. Go to them right away.

4. *Stand close to the child's bed and assure him or her that you will be there.*

When you go to the child's room, stand close to the bed and say "I'm here." **However, do not get into the bed.** Your presence should help alleviate the child's concern and fear of being awake at night with no one else awake, without needing to get into his or her bed. If you have previously made the mistake of sleeping in the child's bed when he or she wakes up, it may take a while for the child to be comfortable with this new arrangement. There may be some initial crying, but you need to avoid getting into the bed.

5. *As your child closes his or her eyes, quietly move back a few steps.*

When you see your child nodding to sleep, move back a few steps. Continue moving away from your child's bed as you see that she or he is falling asleep. Eventually, you will be out of the room. If the child awakens during this process, move back to his or her room and assure the child that you were there and will stay there until she or he falls asleep. However, do not get in their bed! Eventually, you will be able to go back to your bed once they fall into deep sleep.

6. *With next awakening, stay a few steps further away from the bed.*

If your child wakes up a second time during the night, follow the same process, except you should be one or two steps further away from the bed than you were the first time.

7. *Each successive awakening results in you being further away.*

Eventually, you should be able to hear your child call out for you, and you can respond from your bed, "I'm up until you fall asleep." The length of time it will take to get to this point varies by family. Realize that through this progressive fading of your presence, your child has become more and more comfortable with just hearing your voice and not seeing you.

8. *Keep a journal for the first one to two weeks, delineating how the plan went each night.*

You can write in your journal (see sample below) in the morning about how many times your child awoke and how much progress is being made.

Parent Journal of Treatment Progress:
Nighttime Waking

Date: Entry:

Date: Entry:

Date: Entry:

Date: Entry:

Date: Entry:

Date: Entry:

Date: Entry:

Nighttime accidents

1. *Prerequisites to nighttime toileting.*

Your child should be capable of daytime toileting, with minimal or no accidents occurring for a period of weeks. If your child is not toilet trained to a sufficient level, you should implement daytime toileting first before tackling nighttime accidents.

1. *When is your child eliminating at night?*

Prior to any formal strategy, it is necessary to establish the pattern of your child's nighttime eliminations. This is called collecting baseline information. To accomplish this, you will designate three to five "checkpoints" in which you will check your child while she is sleeping to determine if she has had an accident. This definitely needs to be recorded on a nighttime accident data sheet. For example, you might schedule three checkpoints at 10 PM, 12:30 AM, and 3 AM. Do this for least 10 -15 nights, to get an estimate of your child's nighttime pattern.

2. *Teaching your child to awaken at night.*

You should waken your child to go to the toilet about 15 minutes before the checkpoint. You may have to adjust this awakening schedule if you see that the bed is usually wet when you awaken your child. The premise is to catch them before they are usually eliminating and teaching them to wake up and eliminate in the toilet. Have your child go to the toilet and sit for least 5 to 8 minutes. If your child eliminates in the toilet, provide praise, clean your child and send her or him back to the bed. If your child does not eliminate quickly while on the toilet, have your child stay on the toilet until eight minutes have elapsed. Do this for each of the impending checkpoints during the night. Again it is necessary to record both accidents, which involves eliminating in the bed prior to being awakened as well as eliminations in the toilet. You can still use the nighttime accident data sheet.

3. *Teaching your child to self awaken.*

Once you start to see that your child is waking up ahead of your prompt, you can start delaying the awake process by waiting 15 to 20 minutes from the initial time. Tell them before bedtime that if they wake up, they can call out and let you know they are going to the bathroom. Certainly provide praise and an additional incentive for toilet eliminations. You would use the nighttime accident data sheet to record an elimination that occurred independently.

4. *Develop a star chart for "accident free" nights.*

For each night your child is accident free, and eliminates at least one time during the night, he or she should receive a star. You can use the star chart to provide a reward contingent upon earning a designated number of stars, for example, six stars earns a preferred video rental.

5. *Once your child has been successful, you can remove the checkpoints.*

Depending on your child's age, at a point where she is accident free for several nights, you can remove the checkpoints and just allow her to wake up on her own. Continue using the star chart. If accidents become prevalent for several days in a row, go back to step #4 above.

Nighttime Accidents Star Chart:

If child did not have an accident that night, place a star the following morning on that date

SUN	MON	TUES	WED	THURS	FRI	SAT
Date:	Date:	Date:	Date:	Date:	Date:	Date:
Date:	Date:	Date:	Date:	Date:	Date:	Date:
Date:	Date:	Date:	Date:	Date:	Date:	Date:
Date:	Date:	Date:	Date:	Date:	Date:	Date:

Sibling rivalry at home

1. *Plan breaks from each other.*

When children play or interact together, the possibility of arguments and fights exists. The longer they play together, the greater the likelihood of arguments and fights. It is therefore important to realize that in some cases, children may need a break from each other. Sometimes absence makes the heart grow fonder! If they are spending all day together, and every day together, it might not be a bad idea to plan some periods where they play independently. This will not solve the problem completely, but should help out to some degree.

2. *Be Vigilant!*

Be on the lookout for potential conflict! If you are usually catching the argument way after the blows have been struck, then increased vigilance on your part is paramount. You should be aware of what your children are doing, i.e., an open-ear for sounds that appear to be headed for an argument. Your vigilance to potential escalating arguments is vital.

3. *Adopt the Mommy-court approach to disputes regarding items or toys..*

Many arguments and fights with children are over two (or more) of them wanting the same item or toy at the same time. While we would like for our children to learn to share, leaving them to work out the solution to this problem usually leads to arguments and fights. The best way to teach them to share is to have them bring their case to the judge (you) before it comes to blows. This is how it proceeds. At the start of a dispute the children are taught to come to you (the judge) with their complaint regarding the toy in question. Get an oven timer and set it for a small length of time, allowing one child to have that item first. Your other child gets it after the timer goes off, for the same length of time. The child who had the toy first must part with it willingly. If the child who gets it first stops playing with the toy before the timer is up, the second child may get the toy at that time.

4. *Aggression should always result in the aggressor(s) not getting the toy (and time-out removal).*

Once you have given your children a more acceptable way to resolve their disputes and they fail to resort to such, the consequence should be loss of the desired toy for some specified period of time. Arguments and aggression should result in the children's inability to get the desired toy in the immediate future. This would require a removal from the play area for a brief time out, in addition to loss of access to the preferred item for a designated period of time.

5. *Solving disputes via Mommy-court should be praised and reinforced.*

If arguing and fighting are to decrease dramatically, then teaching your children to come to you to solve a dispute in a fair and equitable manner is necessary. Therefore, implementing a point system (along with praise) when they come to the Mommy-court is strongly advised. Each child who comes to the parent to solve a dispute and then abides by the ruling should be reinforced. Keep track of this information in a journal format.

6. *Physical aggression should result in a more significant consequence.*

If the children hit each other, you might consider the loss of a privilege or early bedtime that day as a consequence for the transgressor(s). Here is a real case example. Cesar (not real name), a seven-year-old boy, was referred to me for behavioral services as a result of his mother's request to receive help to control his aggression to his younger brother. Like many siblings arguments occur, but his mother felt she could not control his aggression towards his brother and was worried about it someday getting out of hand. His mother felt that now was the time to extinguish such a behavioral pattern from his repertoire.

After collecting a base rate of aggressive behavior, we designed a plan of action. The plan we designed incorporated both usual bedtime and TV access during prime time as earned privileges. Each aggressive incident toward his sibling would result in one strike. When Cesar reached two strikes, he went to bed one hour early that night (effectively missing all his favorite prime time shows). Cesar did not go to bed early for the first three weeks of the plan. Subsequently, his mother and I agreed to reduce the cut-off to one strike. Cesar continued to succeed on the plan (read Section IV in free downloadable ebook, *Punishment on Trial*, for further information on arranging consequences).

**Parent Journal of Treatment
Progress:**
Sibling Rivalry

Date: Entry:

___

Date: Entry:

___

Date: Entry:

___

Date: Entry:

___

Date: Entry:

___

Date: Entry:

___

Date: Entry:

___

Date: Entry:

Car trips
(The Cipani Tolerance Training Method)

1. *Develop child tolerance of car trips gradually and progressively.*

Especially for young children, relatively lengthy car trips are often not fun. Additionally, being required to be in a child-safety seat (or seat belt) adds additional burden to the aversive nature of car trips. If your child has extreme difficulty staying in his/her seat belt during car trips of varying lengths of time, it might be necessary to gradually develop his/her tolerance gradually. I would suggest having a one to two week training program to teach your child how to ride in the car in his or her car seat. Start with short trips. For example, conduct a car trip around the block. Short and sweet, right? But have several of these trips a day even though there is no purpose to the trip, other than a practice session. By conducting practice sessions, your child has the frequent opportunity to begin to tolerate the situations inherent in car trips, albeit for a short duration. Going back to a preferred play activity following a successful practice session is a good idea.

2. *Gradually increase length of car trips.*

As your child gets better at tolerating trips that last a few minutes, you can progressively expand the length of the trip by increasing the distance driven. Do this gradually over the two week training phase of the program. Don't jump from a two-minute car trip to half an hour! Once your child is capable of car trips involving 10 or 15 minutes, or longer, you and your child will have a more pleasant experience traveling about during your weekly community activities.

3. *Have an alternative activity available to reduce periods of boredom.*

Even during training sessions, bring entertaining materials and activities for your child to engage in. Doing something entertaining and distracting during car trips can be of extreme help when longer trips are necessary. If the child is kept busy, the likelihood of problem behavior during the trip is less.

4. *Be Patient.*

Realize that not every child responds in the same time frame to these suggestions. I suggest that during the training program (first two weeks), several short car trips occur each day. Subsequent to the training program use these suggestions during "real" car trips. Once the child is capable of tolerating reasonable car trips, (i.e., the length of your usual trips), you can fade out the training program. Remember, right now, your children would have a tough time with two-hour car trips irrespective of the training program you have. But with progressive tolerance training, your child can become more manageable with your usual trips to the store, park, Laundromat, etc. Good luck!

Following rules of playground

1. Preview rules before going to playground.

Your rules for the playground should be a short list, so that they easily fit on one index card. The younger the child, the shorter the list (especially in the beginning). You can always add to the list once your child has learned how to respect your initial few rules. Also it is probably advisable to have shorter lengths of time on the playground in the beginning. This facilitates getting your child used to leaving the playground appropriately because of a greater number of opportunities to do so.

2. The consequence for breaking a rule is an immediate brief removal.

If your child breaks a rule, immediately go to your child, indicate what rule they broke and provide a brief removal from the playground area.

3. Set a limit on breaking rules.

On some days, it may seem that your child is forever testing you and the rules. There needs to be a point at which the playground experience is terminated as a consequence of such behavior. Therefore, tell your child that if you have to remove him more than a certain number of times, the playground activity will be immediately terminated. For example, if you designate that three removals is the limit, the following would occur. The first time your child broke a rule, he would simply be removed for a short period of time out. The same would happen for the second time. However, with the third rule violation, the playground experience is ended immediately and you both proceed to go home.

4. When it is over, it is over!

Whether it is an early departure (due to behavior) or the scheduled ending of the play activity, when you say, "It is time to go," that is it. Tell your child he has to the count of five to come to you. If he complies, I would suggest giving him a monetary reward (read Section IV in free downloadable ebook, Punishment on Trial, for further information on arranging consequences). Depending on the age of the child, a dime to a quarter can add up across several weeks. If the child does not comply and either ignores you and engages in tantrums, immediately physically take her away from the playground, with no monetary reward. You might also designate an additional consequence that day for failing to follow your directive to leave the playground, e.g., early bedtime, loss of TV programs, etc.

Putting up toys after play The "Cipani 3 Toy Rule"

1. Have a place where toys are stored.

Does your child have a designated place where to put toys when she or he is done playing with them? Before your child can do his or her part, you must do yours. Toys should be stored in a designated area, either in bins, or where appropriate, on shelves. In other words, there must be a place for each toy.

2. The "Cipani 3-toy" rule!

Don't let your child drag out every toy and then expect that he or she will pick them up when the play activity is concluded! The Cipani 3-toy rule: No more than three toys out at one time. If your child desires a different toy, then he or she must put away one toy to take its place. Pretty simple, but the toil is in your follow-through. When the play activity ends, all of the toys (three or less) must be put up. You can set a timer for the cleanup. If the child does not have the toys cleaned up in the delineated period of time for cleanup, then some time is taken off the next play period to practice; "how to put up toys."

3. Have defined play periods.

It is much easier to monitor the "Cipani 3-toy" rule if they are defined play activities, especially in the beginning. This requires that you designate the play activity schedule. I recommend this to any parent who has difficulty following the "Cipani 3-toy" rule.

Interrupting others during conversations (phone or face to face)

1. *Provide a signal or instruction to your child.*

In order for your child to begin to learn when it is not appropriate to interrupt, a signal and/or instruction indicating that interruptions are not permissible is needed at the beginning of the conversation. A brief verbal explanation, such as, "I will be on the phone with Uncle Henry for the next 4 minutes. Please do not interrupt me until I am finished unless it is an emergency," should suffice.

2. *Delineate the length of time your conversation will entail.*

Letting your child know how long you will be tied up is important. I recommend an oven timer to clearly delineate the length of time your child must go without interruption. Upon initiating the conversation, set the oven timer for the designated length of time and show it to your child. The oven timer is kept in plain view so that your child can see the time left when desired. Once the oven timer goes off, terminate the conversation shortly, or allow your child an opportunity to interrupt briefly and/or participate.

3. *Please use an oven timer for this behavioral strategy.*

The reason for the great reliance on the oven timer is that many children cannot **wait** with unpredictable amounts of time. Subsequently, they interrupt your conversation as a mechanism to get you to end the conversation and engage them. An oven timer makes the "wait" requirement specific. In this manner the length of time your child does not interrupt can be programmed progressively for longer and longer periods of time. It also allows for an error correction procedure (delineated in step 6 below) which is highly effective in teaching your child self-control in this area.

4. *Develop a signal that indicates when your child can be allowed to enter into conversation.*

Once your child is capable of waiting a sufficient period of time during your conversations, you can develop their ability to enter into a conversation when it is appropriate. This social grace is fairly difficult to acquire, since the cues are subtle. Therefore, prior to acquiring this subtle distinction, children need a signal which indicates that entering the conversation appropriately is acceptable at this point in time. The signal can be verbal. For example, "O.K. Johnny you have waited patiently to talk, would you like to say something?"

5. *Teach your child that the consequence of interrupting is a delay in getting your attention.*

This can only be done with an **oven timer** (i.e., reliably and systematically). When your child engages in an interruption, you point that out to him/her immediately and concisely, e.g., "You interrupted." No need for a detailed explanation here. Within a split second of that verbal feedback, you then add extra time (determined a priori) to the oven timer and say, "Now you will have to wait longer." Your child learns that interrupting you while on the phone now results in a delay to your attention.

6. *Tolerance training to develop your child's self-control to "wait".*

> To accomplish this, I have used "fake" phone calls. The parent receives multiple phone calls during a training session, with the child being informed of this in advance. The child is told to try to refrain from interrupting until the oven timer sounds and the parent has hung up the phone. The phone call is limited to a short period of time (e.g., **2 minutes**). The use of an oven timer during this training is paramount. Once your child successfully handles 2 minute conversations, without interrupting, the parent can progressively raise the bar (i.e., the standard) to three minutes. You should continue these training sessions for some period of time. Rome was not built in a day!

7. *Try not to change the standard too quickly.*

> Don't go from 2 minutes to 20 minutes in one day, especially with young children. That speedy progression is almost invariably doomed to defeat. Be happy with small successes. You can eventually get to 10 minutes but it might take a few weeks of training sessions. Consider that you may have waited for three years for your child to learn to refrain from interrupting. Given this fact, waiting another three to six weeks is not so bad.

Morning routine for school days

1. *Get your child up at a consistent time.*

In many cases, children who are difficult to awaken in the morning have an inconsistent bedtime schedule. It is possible that a consistent time schedule for going to bed is all that is needed. If going to bed on time is a problem area in and of itself, then you may need to address this problem area first. Ask your physician for the following advice form: Going to bed on time.

2. *A gradual awake procedure may be needed.*

Some children just have difficulty waking up, even with a consistent bedtime schedule. Waking them up abruptly often produces behavioral problems right away. In these cases, I have recommended that a clock radio be used. The decibel level of the music can be increased gradually over a ten-minute period, thus providing a progressive awakening of your child. Inform your child each night that you will set the alarm for a certain time, and the music will be very faint at first. Once the alarm goes off, you will alter the volume a "notch" every few minutes. After several changes in the volume, your child will be expected to get up and turn off the clock radio. This procedure should eventually teach your child to get out of bed with the lower decibel levels of music.

3. *Keep the same schedule of activities.*

Some parents who have difficulty with their child on school days do not have a predictable morning routine. Unfortunately, they allow their child much discretion on what tasks get performed at what times. The result is chaos in the morning! In order for your child to learn a routine for school days, you must develop one. The routine should be invariant until your child is demonstrating the ability to perform the routine without a problem. I would suggest that you print the specific morning activities on a page taped to the child's bathroom wall, for easy reference.

4. *Bathroom activities first.*

I recommend that the first walk in the morning should be to the bathroom. Teach your child that this process of going to the bathroom first is adhered to each morning. If you have several children you will need to "play" with the scheduling problem. You should have a specific list of activities that needs to be completed in the bathroom (posted if necessary). While in the bathroom s/he takes care of all the activities proscribed for that room, e.g., using the toilet, hand washing, brushing teeth, etc. Once your child has successfully completed all the requirements, s/he leaves the bathroom and heads for the bedroom. The same process is carried out, i.e., take care of all the morning activities for that room before leaving the bedroom. Note that this sequence of events does not allow your child to go watch TV, until she is "ready for school." Take away (i.e., remove) the opportunity to play, until all the necessary activities have been completed.

5. *Do not allow your child to engage in a competing activity (e.g., TV watching).*

Your child should not be allowed access to the TV or play station until everything that needs to be taken care of has been. This seems obvious but you would be surprised how often this occurs. It is often the case that a child (who has difficulty) is placed in front of the TV "to wake-up." Other parents use the TV as an interim event to entertain their child until they are ready to deal with them. Realize that this creates a problem when it is time to switch from a pleasurable activity (TV watching) to a markedly less pleasurable activity (getting ready for school). This switching of activities often develops the conditions for tantrums and fights in the morning. Instead of having them watch TV first, use it as the outcome for finishing all tasks on time (see below).

6. *Once your child has performed all the activities except eating, then s/he eats breakfast.*

A good plan is to structure a really tasty breakfast if your child gets all the morning activities done by a designated time in the morning. If they are tardy and procrastinate they may only get toast, particularly since you had to help them get ready instead of making an elaborate breakfast. Obviously, younger children will need help with some of the tasks. Identify those tasks and where on the schedule they occur. This allows your child to complete other activities independently, and getting your help where needed. Your implementation of steps 5 & 6 teach your child a valuable life lesson: work first-- then play!

7. *Some lengthy activities might be scheduled for the previous night.*

If the morning routine is generally hectic in your household, it might be necessary to have some of the child's activities occur the previous night. Bathing/showering is an activity that often is conducted the night before to avoid a time crunch. Similarly, selecting and placing the clothing for the next day, as well as having all materials in the backpack can also be done the night before.

Parent Journal of Treatment Progress:

Morning Routine

Date: Entry:

Date: Entry:

Date: Entry:

Date: Entry:

Date: Entry:

Date: Entry:

Date: Entry:

Date: Entry:

Parent Handouts for each Treatment Package

(can be posted for easy viewing)

Eating too much

1. Control snacking.

2. Designate a child-size portion for each

meal.

3. Slow down the rate of eating.

4. Activity rewards for weight loss (to be worked out with professional).

Going to bed on time

1. Setup a consistent schedule for

bedtime. 2. A pre-bed routine is

necessary.

3. After the bedtime story, no other competing activities should occur in

bed. 4. A bedtime pass is provided if the child gets to bed by the designated
5. A star chart system for adherence is strongly advocated (to be worked out
time.   with professional).

Night waking
(The Cipani Proximity-fading Method)

1. Go to the child immediately, but do not get in his or her bed 2. Stand close

to the child's bed and assure him or her that you will be there. 3. As your

child closes his or her eyes, quietly move back a few steps. 4. With next

awakening, stay a few steps further away from the bed. 5. Each successive

awakening results in you being further away. 6. Keep a journal for the first

one to two weeks.

Nighttime accidents

1. Prerequisites to nighttime toileting. 2. When

is your child eliminating at night? 3. Teaching

your child to awaken at night. 4. Teaching your

child to self awaken. 5. Develop a star chart for

"accident free" nights.
6. Once your child has been successful, you can remove the checkpoints.

Sibling rivalry at home

1. Plan breaks from each

other. 2. Be Vigilant!
3. Adopt the Mommy-court approach to disputes regarding items or toys..

4. Aggression should always result in the aggressor(s) not getting the toy (and time-out removal).

5. Solving disputes via Mommy-court should be praised and reinforced.

6. Physical aggression should result in a more significant consequence (to be worked out with professional).

Car trips
(The Cipani tolerance training method)

1. Develop child tolerance of car trips gradually and

progressively. 2. Gradually increase length of car trips.
3. Have an alternative activity available to reduce periods of boredom.

Following rules of playground

1. Preview rules before going to playground.

2. The consequence for breaking a rule is an immediate brief

removal. 3. Set a limit on breaking rules.
4. When it is over, it is over!

Putting up toys after play

The "Cipani 3 toy rule"

1. Have a place where toys are

stored. 2. The "Cipani 3-toy" rule!
3. Have defined play periods.

Interrupting others during
conversations
(phone or face to face)

1. Provide a signal or instruction to your child. 2. Delineate

the length of time your conversation will entail. 3. Please

use an oven timer for this behavioral strategy.
4. Develop a signal that indicates when your child can be allowed to enter into
conversation.

5. Teach your child that the consequence of interrupting is a delay in getting
your attention.

6. Tolerance training to develop your child's self-control to

"wait". 7. Try not to change the standard too quickly.

Morning routine for school days

1. Get your child up at a consistent time. 2. A

gradual awake procedure may be needed. 3.

Keep the same schedule of activities. 4.

Bathroom activities first.
5. Do not allow your child to engage in a competing activity

6. Once your child has performed all the activities except eating, then s/he eats
    breakfast.

7. Some lengthy activities might be scheduled for the previous night.

www.ingramcontent.com/pod-product-compliance
Lightning Source LLC
Chambersburg PA
CBHW071007180526
45168CB00003B/1320